The Mind Diet Cookbook for Seniors

The Ultimate 21-Day Meal Plan for a Sharper Brain to Fight Alzheimer's Disease and Dementia

"The Mind Diet Cookbook for Seniors" to nourish both body and mind with specially curated recipes and insights for promoting cognitive wellness.

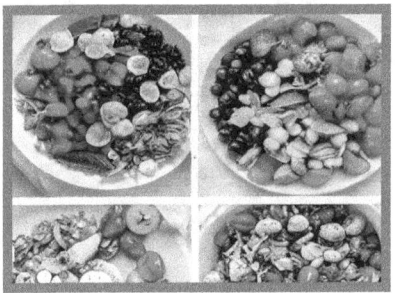

Evelyn Ball

Copyright © 2023 Evelyn Ball

Here is the author's additional book collection

Scan the QR Code Below

Table of Contents

Introduction

Meet Flora and Craig, a loving couple in their golden years who faced an unexpected challenge of Alzheimer's disease. Their journey was filled with uncertainties, but they refused to let it define their lives. Instead, they embarked on a mission to reclaim their health and happiness through the power of nutrition.

In their quest, they discovered the "Mind Diet Cookbook for Seniors," a remarkable guide that would forever alter the course of their battle. This cookbook wasn't just about recipes; it was a lifeline, a source of hope. With each carefully crafted dish, Flora and Craig nurtured their bodies and minds, promoting mental clarity and well-being.

Their story is a testament to the transformative potential of food, proving that a nourishing diet tailored for Alzheimer's can be a powerful ally in the fight against cognitive decline. As you explore the pages of this cookbook, you'll uncover the very recipes that brought light back into Flora and Craig's lives. Together, let's embark on a journey to better health and a brighter future, one delicious meal at a time.

Understanding Alzheimer's and Nutrition

What You Should Know

Alzheimer's disease is a condition that affects the brain, causing problems with memory and thinking. While there's no cure, what you eat can make a big difference.

The Link Between Diet and Cognitive Health

Some diets, like the Mediterranean diet, seem to protect against Alzheimer's. They include lots of fruits, veggies, whole grains, lean protein (like chicken), and healthy fats (like olive oil). These foods have special nutrients that help keep your brain working well.

Nutritional Guidelines for Alzheimer's

If you or someone you know has Alzheimer's, here are some tips:

1. **Balance Diet:** This gives your brain all the nutrients it needs.

2. **Omega -3 fatty acid:** Try to eat fish like salmon and foods with flax seeds. They have things that are good for your brain.

3. **Antioxidants:** fruits and veggies with bright colors like blueberries and spinach. They help protect your brain.

4. **Stay away from sugary and processed foods.** They can make your brain work worse.

5. **Hydration:** Drink enough water because even being a little thirsty can make your brain work badly.

6. **Portions Control:** eat too much at once. Eating big meals can make you feel uncomfortable.

7. **Regular Meal:** at regular times. It can make you feel safer and more relaxed.

8. **Consult Healthcare Professional:** Ask a doctor or dietitian for help. They can make a food plan just for you.

So, what you eat really matters when it comes to Alzheimer's. It can help you think better and feel better, too!

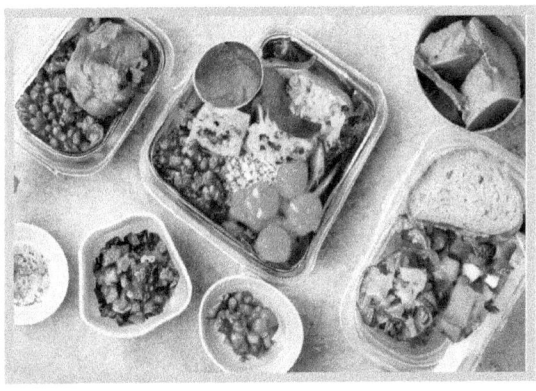

Week 1: Day 1

Boosting Brain Health

Breakfast

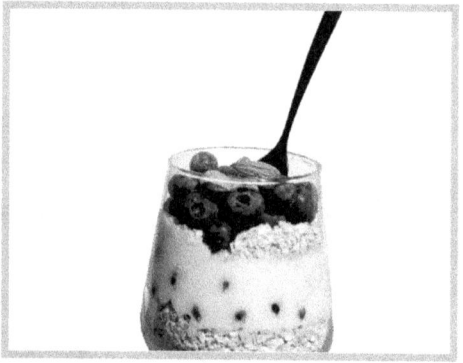

Greek Yogurt Parfait

- **Preparation Time: 5 minutes**

- **Ingredients:**

- 1/2 cup Greek yogurt

- 1/4 cup granola

- One-fourth cup of mixed berries (strawberries, blueberries).

- 1 tablespoon honey

- **Directions:**

1. In a glass, layer Greek yogurt, granola, and mixed berries.

2. Drizzle honey over the top.

Nutrition Value per Serving: Calories: 250 kcal | Protein: 10g | Carbs: 35g | Fat: 8g | Fiber: 5g

Lunch

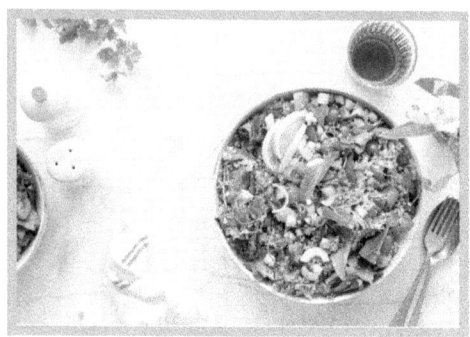

Quinoa salad with chickpeas and vegetables

- Preparation Time: 15 minutes

- Ingredients:

- 1/2 cup cooked quinoa

- 1/4 cup washed and drained canned chickpeas

- 1/4 cup diced cucumber

- 1/4 cup diced bell peppers

- 2 tablespoons diced red onion

- 2 tablespoons feta cheese, crumbled

- 2 tablespoons lemon juice

- 1 tablespoon olive oil

- Fresh parsley for garnish

- Salt and pepper to taste.

Directions:

1. In a bowl, combine quinoa, chickpeas, cucumber, bell peppers, red onion, and feta cheese.

2. Drizzle with lemon juice and olive oil. Season with salt and pepper.

3. Garnish with fresh parsley.

Nutrition Value per Serving: Calories: 300 kcal | Protein: 12g | Carbs: 35g | Fat: 12g | Fiber: 6g

Dinner

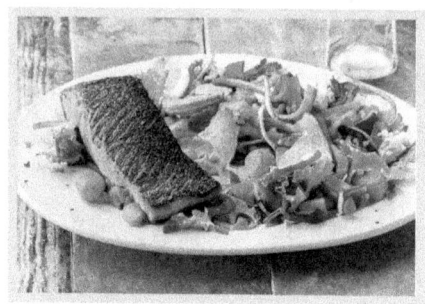

Baked Salmon with Roasted Vegetables

- Preparation Time: 30 minutes

- Ingredients:

- 4 oz salmon fillet

- 1/2 cup broccoli florets

- 1/2 cup diced carrots

- 1/4 cup diced bell peppers

- 1 tablespoon olive oil

- 1 teaspoon dried herbs (oregano, thyme)

- Lemon wedges for serving

- Salt and pepper to taste

- Directions:

1. Preheat the oven. Place salmon on a baking sheet.

2. Toss broccoli, carrots, and bell peppers with olive oil and dried herbs.

3. Spread vegetables around salmon. Season everything with salt and pepper.

4. Bake until salmon is cooked through and vegetables are tender.

5. Serve with lemon wedges.

Nutrition Value per Serving: Calories: 350 kcal | Protein: 25g | Carbs: 15g | Fat: 20g | Fiber: 5g

Snack

Apple Slices with Almond Butter

- Preparation Time: 5 minutes

- Ingredients:

- 1 medium apple, sliced

- 2 tablespoons almond butter

- Directions:

1. Dip apple slices in almond butter.

- Nutrition Value per Serving:

Calories: 200 kcal

Protein: 4g

Carbs: 25g

Fat: 10g

Fiber: 6g

Week 1: Day 2

Breakfast

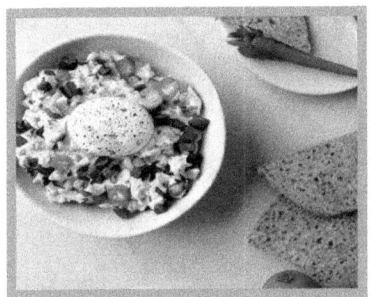

Scrambled Eggs with Spinach and Feta

- **Preparation Time: 10 minutes**

- **Ingredients:**

  - 2 eggs

  - 1/4 cup fresh spinach, chopped

  - 2 tablespoons crumbled feta cheese

  - 1 teaspoon olive oil

  - Salt and pepper to taste

- Directions:

1. In a bowl, whisk eggs with spinach and feta cheese.

2. Heat olive oil in a pan. Pour in egg mixture and scramble until cooked.

3. Season with salt and pepper.

- Nutrition Value per Serving: Calories: 250 kcal | Protein: 18g | Carbs: 4g | Fat: 18g | Fiber: 1g

Lunch

Mediterranean Hummus Wrap

- Preparation Time: 10 minutes

- Ingredients:

- 1 whole-grain pasta tortilla or wrap

- 1/4 cup hummus

- 1/4 cup diced cucumbers

- 1/4 cup diced tomatoes

- 2 tablespoons chopped kalamata olives

- 2 tablespoons crumbled feta cheese

- Fresh parsley for garnish

- Directions:

1. Lay out wrap. Spread hummus evenly over the surface.

2. Layer cucumbers, tomatoes, kalamata olives, and feta cheese.

3. Garnish with fresh parsley.

4. Roll up tightly and enjoy.

- Nutrition Value per Serving: Calories: 300 kcal | Protein: 10g | Carbs: 35g | Fat: 15g | Fiber: 8g

Dinner

Grilled Chicken with Lemon-Herb Quinoa

- Preparation Time: 40 minutes

- Ingredients:

- 4 ounces of skinless, boneless chicken breast

- 1/2 cup cooked quinoa

- Zest and juice of 1 lemon

- 1 tablespoon of freshly harvested herbs, chopped (thyme, rosemary)

- 1 teaspoon olive oil

- Salt and pepper to taste

- Directions:

1. Preheat the grill. Season chicken with lemon zest, chopped herbs, olive oil, salt, and pepper.

2. Grill chicken until cooked through.

3. In a bowl, mix cooked quinoa with lemon juice.

4. Serve grilled chicken over lemon-herb quinoa.

- **Nutrition Value per Serving:** Calories: 320 kcal | Protein: 30g | Carbs: 25g | Fat: 10g | Fiber: 4g

Snack

Mixed Nuts

- **Preparation Time: 5 minutes**

- **Ingredients:**

   - 1/4 cup mixed nuts (almonds, walnuts, pistachios)

- **Directions:**

1. Enjoy a handful of mixed nuts as a snack.

- **Nutrition Value per Serving:** Calories: 200 kcal | Protein: 6g | Carbs: 6g

| Fat: 18g | Fiber: 3g

Week 1: Day 3

Breakfast

Oatmeal with Berries and Almonds

- Preparation Time: 10 minutes

- Ingredients:

- 1/2 cup oats

- 1 cup water or milk (dairy or plant-based)

- 1/4 cup mixed berries (blueberries, raspberries)

- 1 tablespoon chopped almonds

- 1 teaspoon honey

- Directions:

1. Cook oats with water or milk according to package instructions.

2. Top with mixed berries, chopped almonds, and a drizzle of honey.

- **Nutrition Value per Serving:** Calories: 280 kcal | Protein: 8g | Carbs: 40g | Fat: 10g | Fiber: 6g

Lunch

Spinach Salad with Grilled Shrimp

- **Preparation Time: 20 minutes**

- **Ingredients:**

  - 4 ounces of separated and deveined shrimp

  - 2 cups fresh spinach leaves

  - 1/4 cup cherry tomatoes, halved

  - 1/4 cup sliced cucumbers

  - 1/4 avocado, sliced

  - 2 tablespoons balsamic vinaigrette

- **Directions:**

  1. Preheat the grill. Season shrimp and grill until cooked.

2. In a bowl, combine spinach, cherry tomatoes, cucumbers, and avocado.

3. Top with grilled shrimp and drizzle with balsamic vinaigrette.

- **Nutrition Value per Serving:** Calories: 250 kcal | Protein: 20g | Carbs: 15g | Fat: 12g | Fiber: 6g

Dinner

Mediterranean Baked Cod

- Preparation Time: 30 minutes

- Ingredients:

- 4 oz cod fillet

- 1/4 cup diced tomatoes

- 1/4 cup diced red onion

- 2 tablespoons chopped Kalamata olives

- 1 tablespoon chopped fresh parsley

- 1 tablespoon olive oil

- Lemon wedges for serving

- Salt and pepper to taste

- Directions:

1. Preheat the oven. Cod fillet should be put on a baking pan.

2. Top with diced tomatoes, red onion, Kalamata olives, and chopped parsley.

3. Sprinkle salt and pepper over top and drizzle with olive oil.

4. Bake until the cod is cooked through.

5. Serve with lemon wedges.

- Nutrition Value per Serving: Calories: 220 kcal | Protein: 25g | Carbs: 8g | Fat: 10g | Fiber: 2g

Snack

Carrot and Hummus

- **Preparation Time: 5 minutes**

- **Ingredients**:

  - 1 medium carrot, sliced

  - 2 tablespoons hummus

Directions:

1. Dip carrot slices in hummus.

Nutrition Value per Serving: Calories: 150 kcal | Protein: 4g | Carbs: 18g | Fat: 8g | Fiber: 5g

Week 1: Day 4

Breakfast

Greek Yogurt with Walnuts and Honey

- **Preparation Time: 5 minutes**

- **Ingredients:**

  - 1/2 cup Greek yogurt

  - 2 tablespoons chopped walnuts

  - 1 teaspoon honey

- **Directions:**

  1. In a bowl, combine Greek yogurt and chopped walnuts.

  2. Drizzle with honey.

- Nutrition Value per Serving: Calories: 250 kcal | Protein: 10g | Carbs: 10g | Fat: 18g | Fiber: 2g

Lunch

Caprese Salad

- **Preparation Time: 10 minutes**

- **Ingredients:**

  - 1 large tomato, sliced

  - 1/8 cup thinly sliced fresh mozzarella cheese

  - 1/4 cup fresh basil leaves

  - 1 tablespoon balsamic vinegar

  - 1 tablespoon olive oil

  - Salt and pepper to taste

- **Directions:**

  1. Arrange tomato and mozzarella slices on a plate.

  2. Tuck fresh basil leaves between slices.

  3. Finish by adding olive oil and balsamic vinegar.

  4. Season with salt and pepper.

Nutrition Value per Serving:

Calories: 220 kcal Protein: 10g

Carbs: 5g

Fat: 18g

Fiber: 1g

Dinner

Stuffed Bell Peppers

- Preparation Time: 40 minutes

- Ingredients:

- 1/2 cup cooked lean ground turkey and two bell peppers that have been cut in half and their seeds removed

- 1/4 cup cooked quinoa

- 1/4 cup diced tomatoes

- 1/4 cup diced zucchini

- 2 tablespoons shredded mozzarella cheese

- 1 tablespoon olive oil

- 1/2 teaspoon Italian seasoning

- Salt and pepper to taste

- Directions:

1. Preheat the oven. Put the halves of the bell pepper in a baking dish.

2. In a bowl, mix ground turkey, cooked quinoa, diced tomatoes, diced zucchini, mozzarella cheese, olive oil, Italian seasoning, salt, and pepper.

3. Fill bell pepper halves with the mixture.

4. Bake until peppers are tender and filling is heated through.

- Nutrition Value per Serving: Calories: 300 kcal | Protein: 20g | Carbs: 20g | Fat: 15g | Fiber: 4g

Snack

Cottage Cheese with Pineapple

- **Preparation Time: 5 minutes**

- **Ingredients:**

  - 1/2 cup low-fat cottage cheese

  - 1/4 cup diced pineapple

- Directions:

  1. Combine cottage cheese and diced pineapple in a bowl.

- **Nutrition Value per Serving:** Calories: 180 kcal | Protein: 15g | Carbs: 20g | Fat: 5g | Fiber: 2g

Week 1: Day 5

Breakfast

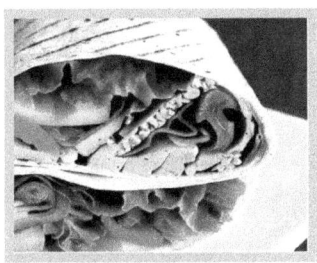

Whole Grain Toast with Avocado

- **Preparation Time: 5 minutes**

- **Ingredients:**

  - 1 toast-flavored slice of whole-grain bread

  - 1/4 avocado, mashed

  - 1 teaspoon lemon juice

  - Red pepper flakes (optional)

- **Directions**:

1. Spread mashed avocado on toasted whole grain bread.

2. Drizzle with lemon juice and sprinkle red pepper flakes if desired.

- **Nutrition Value per Serving:** Calories: 200 kcal | Protein: 5g | Carbs: 20g | Fat: 12g | Fiber: 5g

Lunch

Lentil Soup with Spinach

- **Preparation Time: 30 minutes**

- **Ingredients:**

  - 1/2 cup dried green lentils, rinsed and drained

  - 2 cups vegetable broth

  - 1/4 cup diced carrots

  - 1/4 cup diced celery

  - 1/4 cup diced onion

- 1 cup fresh spinach leaves

- 1 teaspoon olive oil

- 1/2 teaspoon cumin

- Salt and pepper to taste

- Directions:

1. In a pot, heat olive oil. Add diced carrots, celery, and onion. Sauté until tender.

2. Add lentils, vegetable broth, cumin, salt, and pepper. Lentils should be cooked for a minimum of 20 minutes at a simmer.

3. Stir in fresh spinach leaves and cook until wilted.

- Nutrition Value per Serving: Calories: 250 kcal | Protein: 15g | Carbs: 40g | Fat: 4g | Fiber: 15g

Dinner

Grilled Vegetable Salad

- **Preparation Time: 20 minutes**

- **Ingredients:**

    - 1 cup mixed grilled vegetables (zucchini, bell peppers, eggplant)

    - 1/4 cup cooked quinoa

    - 2 cups mixed greens

    - 2 tablespoons balsamic vinaigrette

    - 1 tablespoon crumbled goat cheese

- **Directions:**

    1. Toss mixed grilled vegetables with cooked quinoa and mixed greens.

    2. Drizzle with balsamic vinaigrette and top with crumbled goat cheese.

- **Nutrition Value per Serving:** Calories: 280 kcal | Protein: 8g | Carbs: 35g | Fat: 12g | Fiber: 8g

Snack

Rice Cakes with Almond Butter

- **Preparation Time: 5 minutes**

- **Ingredients:**

  - 2 rice cakes

  - 2 tablespoons almond butter

- **Directions:**

  1. Spread almond butter on rice cakes.

- Nutrition Value per Serving: Calories: 220 kcal | Protein: 6g | Carbs: 25g | Fat: 12g | Fiber: 3g

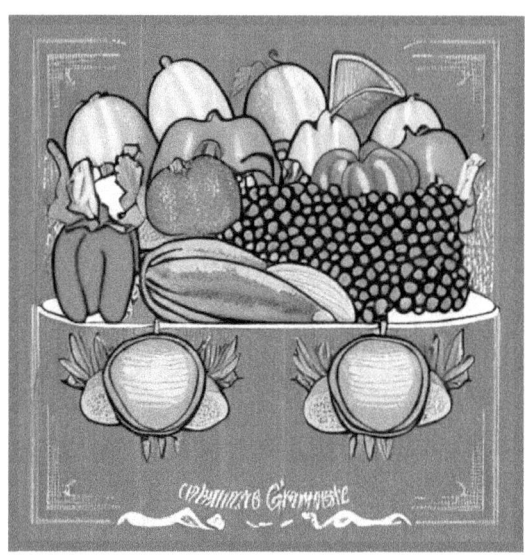

Week 1: Day 6

Breakfast

Smoothie with Mixed Berries

- **Preparation Time: 5 minutes**

- **Ingredients:**

Berry mixture of blueberries, raspberries, and strawberries, 1/2 cup

- 1/2 banana

- 1/2 cup unsweetened almond milk

- 1/4 cup Greek yogurt

- 1 tablespoon chia seeds

- 1 teaspoon honey

- **Directions:**

1. Blend mixed berries, banana, almond milk, Greek yogurt, and chia seeds until smooth.

2. Drizzle with honey.

- **Nutrition Value per Serving:** Calories: 250 kcal | Protein: 8g | Carbs: 40g | Fat: 8g | Fiber: 10g.

Lunch

Tuna Salad Lettuce Wraps

- **Preparation Time: 15 minutes**

- **Ingredients:**

  - 1 can (5 oz) tuna in water, drained

  - 2 tablespoons Greek yogurt

  - 1 tablespoon Dijon mustard

  - 1/4 cup diced celery

  - 1/4 cup diced red onion

  - Lettuce leaves for wrapping

  - Salt and pepper to taste

Directions:

1. In a bowl, mix tuna, Greek yogurt, Dijon mustard, diced celery, and red onion.

2. Season with salt and pepper.

3. Spoon tuna mixture onto lettuce leaves and wrap.

- **Nutrition Value per Serving:** Calories: 220 kcal | Protein: 25g | Carbs: 10g | Fat: 8g | Fiber: 2g

Dinner

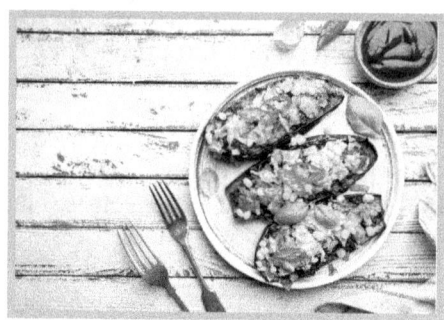

Baked Eggplant Parmesan

- Preparation Time: 45 minutes

- Ingredients:

- 1 small eggplant, sliced

- 1/4 cup whole wheat breadcrumbs

- 1/4 cup grated Parmesan cheese

- 1/2 cup marinara sauce (low-sodium)

- 1/4 cup shredded mozzarella cheese

- Fresh basil leaves for garnish

- Olive oil cooking spray

- Salt and pepper to taste

- **Directions:**

1. Preheat the oven. Spread olive oil cooking spray on slices of eggplant.

2. Combine breadcrumbs, grated Parmesan cheese, salt, and pepper.

3. Coat eggplant slices with breadcrumb mixture and place on a baking sheet.

4. Bake until the eggplant is tender and the coating is golden.

5. In a baking dish, layer baked eggplant slices, marinara sauce, and shredded mozzarella cheese. Repeat layers.

6. Bake until the cheese is melted and bubbly.

7. Garnish with fresh basil leaves.

- **Nutrition Value per Serving:** Calories: 320 kcal | Protein: 15g | Carbs: 30g | Fat: 15g | Fiber: 10g.

Snack

Yogurt with Berries

- **Preparation Time: 5 minutes**

- **Ingredients:**

  - 1/2 cup plain Greek yogurt

  - 1/4 cup mixed berries (blueberries, raspberries)

  - 1 teaspoon honey

- **Directions:**

  1. In a bowl, mix Greek yogurt with mixed berries.

  2. Drizzle with honey.

- Nutrition Value per Serving: Calories: 150 kcal | Protein: 15g | Carbs: 20g | Fat: 2g | Fiber: 4g

Week 1: Day 7

Breakfast

Almond Butter Banana Toast

- Preparation Time: 5 minutes

- Ingredients:

- 1 toast-flavored slice of whole-grain bread

- 1 tablespoon almond butter

- 1/2 banana, sliced

- Directions:

1. Spread almond butter on toasted whole grain bread.

2. Top with banana slices.

Nutrition Value per Serving: Calories: 250 kcal | Protein: 6g | Carbs: 30g | Fat: 12g | Fiber: 5g

Lunch

Mediterranean Chickpea Salad

- Preparation Time: 15 minutes

- Ingredients:

- A can of chickpeas that have been cleaned and drained

- 1/4 cup diced cucumber

- 1/4 cup red bell peppers, diced

- 1/4 cup diced red onion

- 1/4 cup chopped fresh parsley

- 2 tablespoons feta cheese, crumbled

- 1 tablespoon olive oil

- 1 tablespoon lemon juice

- Salt and pepper to taste

- Directions:

1. In a bowl, combine chickpeas, cucumber, red bell pepper, red onion, parsley, and feta cheese.

2. Garnish with lemon juice and olive oil. Season with salt and pepper.

- Nutrition Value per Serving: Calories: 280 kcal | Protein: 12g | Carbs: 35g | Fat: 10g | Fiber: 8g

Dinner

Roasted Chicken with Mediterranean Vegetables

- Preparation Time: 50 minutes

- Ingredients:

- 4 ounces of skinless, boneless chicken breast

- 1/2 cup diced zucchini

- 1/2 cup diced eggplant

- 1/4 cup diced red onion

- 1/4 cup cherry tomatoes, halved

- 2 tablespoons olive oil

- 1 teaspoon dried oregano

- 1 teaspoon lemon juice

- Salt and pepper to taste

Directions:

1. Preheat the oven. Toss zucchini, eggplant, red onion, and cherry tomatoes with olive oil and dried oregano.

2. Season chicken with lemon juice, salt, and pepper. Place on a baking sheet.

3. Arrange vegetables around chicken. Roast the chicken and veggies until they are both fully done.

- Nutrition Value per Serving: Calories: 350 kcal | Protein: 25g | Carbs: 15g | Fat: 20g | Fiber: 5g

Snack

Mixed Berries Smoothie

- **Preparation Time: 5 minutes**

- **Ingredients:**

    - Berry mixture of blueberries, raspberries, and strawberries, 1/2 cup

    - 1/2 cup unsweetened almond milk

    - 1/4 cup Greek yogurt

    - 1 tablespoon chia seeds

    - 1 teaspoon honey

- **Directions:**

1. Blend mixed berries, almond milk, Greek yogurt, chia seeds, and honey until smooth.

- **Nutrition Value per Serving:** Calories: 180 kcal | Protein: 8g | Carbs: 20g | Fat: 8g | Fiber: 6g

Week 2: Day 8

Nourishing Cognitive Function

Breakfast

Blueberry Chia Seed Pudding

- **Preparation Time: 10 minutes (plus overnight chilling)**

- **Ingredients:**

  - 1/4 cup chia seeds

  - 1 cup unsweetened almond milk

  - 1/2 teaspoon vanilla extract

  - 1/4 cup blueberries

  - 1 tablespoon sliced almonds

- **Directions:**

1. In a bowl, mix chia seeds, almond milk, and vanilla extract.

2. Cover and refrigerate overnight.

3. In the morning, layer chia seed pudding with blueberries and sliced almonds.

- **Nutrition Value per Serving:** Calories: 220 kcal | Protein: 6g | Carbs: 20g | Fat: 14g | Fiber: 10g

Lunch

Grilled Vegetable Wrap

- Preparation Time: 20 minutes

- Ingredients:

- 1 whole wheat tortilla

- 1/2 cup grilled mixed vegetables (zucchini, bell peppers, eggplant)

- 2 tablespoons hummus

- 1/4 cup mixed greens

- 1 tablespoon crumbled feta cheese

- Directions:

1. Spread hummus on the whole wheat tortilla.

2. Top with grilled mixed vegetables, mixed greens, and feta cheese.

3. Roll up the tortilla into a wrap.

- Nutrition Value per Serving: Calories: 250 kcal | Protein: 8g | Carbs: 30g | Fat: 10g | Fiber: 8g.

Dinner

- *Lemon Herb Baked Salmon*

- **Preparation Time: 25 minutes**

- **Ingredients:**

  - 4 oz salmon fillet

  - 1 tablespoon olive oil

  - 1 teaspoon lemon juice

  - 1/2 teaspoon dried dill

  - 1/4 teaspoon garlic powder

  - Lemon slices for garnish

  - Salt and pepper to taste

- **Directions:**

  1. Preheat the oven. Place salmon fillet on a baking sheet.

  2. Drizzle olive oil and lemon juice over the salmon.

3. Sprinkle with dried dill, garlic powder, salt, and pepper.

4. Top with lemon slices.

5. Bake until salmon flakes easily with a fork.

- **Nutrition Value per Serving:** Calories: 300 kcal | Protein: 25g | Carbs: 2g | Fat: 20g | Fiber: 0g

Snack

Carrot Sticks with Hummus

- **Preparation Time: 5 minutes**

- **Ingredients:**

- 1 carrot, cut into sticks

- 2 tablespoons hummus

- **Directions:**

1. Serve carrot sticks with hummus for dipping.

- **Nutrition Value per Serving:** Calories: 100 kcal | Protein: 2g | Carbs: 10g | Fat: 6g | Fiber: 3

Week 2: Day 9

Breakfast

Greek Yogurt Parfait

- **Preparation Time: 10 minutes**

- **Ingredients:**

  - 1/2 cup Greek yogurt

  - 1/4 cup granola

  - a quarter cup of mixed berries (strawberries, blueberries)

  - 1 tablespoon chopped nuts, such as walnuts and almonds

  - Honey for drizzling

- **Directions:**

  1. In a glass, layer Greek yogurt, granola, mixed berries, and chopped nuts.

  2. Drizzle with honey.

- **Nutrition Value per Serving:** Calories: 250 kcal |
Protein: 15g | Carbs: 25g | Fat: 10g | Fiber: 4g

Lunch

Spinach and Feta Stuffed Chicken

- **Preparation Time: 30 minutes**

- **Ingredients:**

  - Unboned, skinless chicken breast weighing 4 ounces

  - 1/4 cup cooked spinach

  - 2 tablespoons crumbled feta cheese

  - 1/4 teaspoon dried oregano

  - Salt and pepper to taste

- **Directions:**

1. Preheat the oven. Butterfly chicken breast and season with salt, pepper, and dried oregano.

2. Stuff with cooked spinach and crumbled feta cheese.

3. Secure with toothpicks.

4. Bake the chicken until it is fully done.

- Nutrition Value per Serving: Calories: 220 kcal | Protein: 30g | Carbs: 2g | Fat: 10g | Fiber: 1g

Dinner

Quinoa Stuffed Bell Peppers

- Preparation Time: 40 minutes

- Ingredients:

- seeds and half-cut bell peppers

- 1/2 cup cooked quinoa

- 1/4 cup washed and drained black beans

- 1/4 cup diced tomatoes

- 1/4 cup diced zucchini

- 2 tablespoons shredded cheddar cheese

- 1 tablespoon chopped fresh cilantro

- 1 teaspoon olive oil

- 1/4 teaspoon ground cumin

- Salt and pepper to taste

Directions:

1. Preheat the oven. Brush bell pepper halves with olive oil and roast until tender.

2. In a bowl, mix cooked quinoa, black beans, diced tomatoes, diced zucchini, shredded cheddar cheese, chopped cilantro, ground cumin, salt, and pepper.

3. Stuffed bell pepper halves with quinoa mixture.

4. Bake until the filling is thoroughly cooked.

- **Nutrition Value per Serving:** Calories: 300 kcal | Protein: 15g | Carbs: 40g | Fat: 10g | Fiber: 8g

Snack

Cottage Cheese with Pineapple

- Preparation Time: 5 minutes

- Ingredients:

  - 1/2 cup low-fat cottage cheese

  - 1/4 cup diced pineapple

- Directions:

  1. Serve cottage cheese with diced pineapple.

- Nutrition Value per Serving: Calories: 150 kcal | Protein: 15g | Carbs: 15g | Fat: 3g | Fiber: 2g

Week 2: Day 10

Breakfast

Oatmeal with Almonds and Berries

- **Preparation Time: 10 minutes**

- **Ingredients:**

  - 1/2 cup rolled oats

  - 1 cup unsweetened almond milk

  - 1 tablespoon chopped almonds

  - 1/4 cup mixed berries (blueberries, raspberries)

  - 1 teaspoon honey

- **Directions:**

  1. Cook rolled oats with almond milk according to package instructions.

  2. Top with chopped almonds, mixed berries, and honey.

- **Nutrition Value per Serving:** Calories: 300 kcal | Protein: 8g | Carbs: 40g | Fat: 10g | Fiber: 6g

Lunch

Tuna and White Bean Salad

- **Preparation Time: 15 minutes**

- **Ingredients:**

  - 1/2 cup canned white beans, drained and rinsed

  - 1/4 cup canned tuna, drained

  - 1/4 cup diced cucumber

  - A quarter cup, chopped red bell peppers

  - 1 tablespoon chopped red onion

  - 1 tablespoon olive oil

  - 1 tablespoon lemon juice

- 1 teaspoon Dijon mustard

- Fresh parsley for garnish

- Salt and pepper to taste

- **Directions:**

1. In a bowl, combine white beans, canned tuna, cucumber, red bell pepper, red onion, chopped parsley, olive oil, lemon juice, Dijon mustard, salt, and pepper.

- **Nutrition Value per Serving:** Calories: 280 kcal | Protein: 20g | Carbs: 25g | Fat: 12g | Fiber: 8g

Dinner

Lentil and Vegetable Stir-Fry

- Preparation Time: 25 minutes

- Ingredients:

- 1/2 cup cooked lentils

- Half a cup of mixed vegetables (carrots, bell peppers, and broccoli)

- 2 tablespoons low-sodium soy sauce

- 1 tablespoon olive oil

- 1/2 teaspoon minced ginger

- 1/4 teaspoon garlic powder

- crushed red pepper flakes equivalent to 1/8 teaspoon

Directions:

1. In a pan, heat olive oil. Combine the vegetables and cook through until tender.

2. Stir in cooked lentils, low-sodium soy sauce, minced ginger, garlic powder, and crushed red pepper flakes.

- Nutrition Value per Serving: Calories: 250 kcal | Protein: 12g | Carbs: 40g | Fat: 5g | Fiber: 10g

Snack

Apple Slices with Peanut Butter

- Preparation Time: 5 minutes

- Ingredients:

- 1 small apple, sliced

- 1 tablespoon natural peanut butter

- Directions:

1. Serve apple slices with peanut butter for dipping.

- Nutrition Value per Serving: Calories: 180 kcal | Protein: 5g | Carbs: 25g | Fat: 8g | Fiber: 5g

Week 2: Day 11

Breakfast

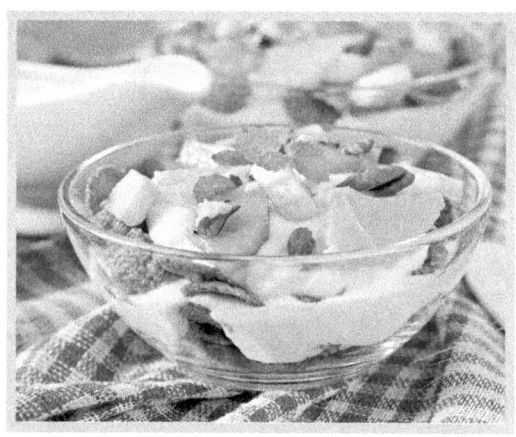

Greek Yogurt with Walnuts and Honey

- Preparation Time: 5 minutes

- Ingredients:

- 1/2 cup Greek yogurt

- 2 tablespoons chopped walnuts

- 1 tablespoon honey

- **Directions**:

1. In a bowl, mix Greek yogurt with chopped walnuts.

2. Drizzle with honey.

- **Nutrition Value per Serving:** Calories: 250 kcal | Protein: 15g | Carbs: 15g | Fat: 15g | Fiber: 2g

Lunch

Caprese Salad

- **Preparation Time: 10 minutes**

- **Ingredients:**

  - 1 medium tomato, sliced

  - 2 ounces of sliced newly harvested mozzarella cheese

  - 1/4 cup fresh basil leaves

  - 1 tablespoon balsamic vinegar

- 1 tablespoon olive oil

- Salt and pepper to taste

- **Directions:**

1. Arrange tomato and mozzarella slices on a plate.

2. Top with fresh basil leaves.

3. Add a drizzle of olive oil and balsamic vinegar.

Nutrition Value per Serving: Calories: 300 kcal | Protein: 10g | Carbs: 5g | Fat: 25g | Fiber: 1g

Dinner

Baked Chicken with Roasted Vegetables

- Preparation Time: 30 minutes

- Ingredients:

- 4 ounces of skinless, boneless chicken breast

- 1/2 cup mixed vegetables (zucchini, bell peppers, onions)

- 1 tablespoon olive oil

- 1/2 teaspoon dried rosemary

- Salt and pepper to taste

- Directions:

1. Preheat the oven. Place chicken breast and mixed vegetables on a baking sheet.

2. Drizzle with olive oil and sprinkle with dried rosemary, salt, and pepper.

3. Bake until chicken is cooked through and vegetables are roasted.

Nutrition Value per Serving:

Calories: 280 kcal

Protein: 25g

Carbs: 10g

Fat: 15g

Fiber: 3g.

Snack

Trail Mix

- **Preparation Time: 5 minutes**

- **Ingredients:**

  - 2 tablespoons mixed nuts (almonds, walnuts)

  - 1 tablespoon dried cranberries

  - 1 tablespoon dark chocolate chips

- **Directions:**

  1. Mix nuts, dried cranberries, and dark chocolate chips.

- **Nutrition Value per Serving:** Calories: 150 kcal | Protein: 4g | Carbs: 10g | Fat: 11g | Fiber: 2g

Week 2: Day 12

Breakfast

- *Banana Oat Pancakes*

- **Preparation Time: 20 minutes**

- **Ingredients:**

  - 1 ripe banana

  - 1/2 cup rolled oats

  - 1/4 cup unsweetened almond milk

  - 1/2 teaspoon vanilla extract

  - 1/2 teaspoon ground cinnamon

  - 1 egg

- **Directions:**

  1. In a blender, combine banana, rolled oats, almond milk, vanilla extract, ground cinnamon, and egg.

2. Blend until smooth.

3. Heat a non-stick pan and pour pancake batter.

4. Cook until bubbles form, then flip and cook until golden.

- Nutrition Value per Serving: Calories: 250 kcal | Protein: 8g | Carbs: 40g | Fat: 6g | Fiber: 6g

Lunch - Mediterranean Chickpea Salad

- Preparation Time: 15 minutes

- Ingredients:

- 1 cup washed and drained canned chickpeas

- 1/4 cup diced cucumber

- 1/4 cup diced tomatoes

- 2 tablespoons chopped red onion

- 2 tablespoons crumbled feta cheese

- 1 tablespoon chopped fresh parsley

- 1 tablespoon olive oil

- 1 tablespoon lemon juice

- 1/2 teaspoon dried oregano

- Salt and pepper to taste

- Directions:

1. In a bowl, combine chickpeas, cucumber, tomatoes, red onion, feta cheese, chopped parsley, olive oil, lemon juice, dried oregano, salt, and pepper.

- Nutrition Value per Serving:

Calories: 280 kcal | Protein: 10g | Carbs: 35g | Fat: 10g | Fiber: 8g

Dinner

Ground turkey-stuffed bell peppers.

- **Preparation Time: 35 minutes**

- **Ingredients:**

  - 2 bell peppers, seeded and cut in half

  - 1/2 cup cooked quinoa

  - 1/4 lb ground turkey

  - 1/4 cup diced tomatoes

  - 1/4 cup diced zucchini

  - 2 tablespoons shredded mozzarella cheese

  - 1 tablespoon chopped fresh basil

  - 1 teaspoon olive oil

  - Salt and pepper to taste

- **Directions:**

  1. Preheat the oven. Brush bell pepper halves with olive oil and roast until tender.

2. In a pan, cook ground turkey until browned. Stir in diced tomatoes, diced zucchini, cooked quinoa, chopped basil, salt, and pepper.

3. Stuffed bell pepper halves with the turkey mixture.

4. Top with shredded mozzarella cheese.

5. Bake until the cheese is melted and golden.

- **Nutrition Value per Serving:** Calories: 320 kcal

| Protein: 20g | Carbs: 25g | Fat: 15g | Fiber: 6g

Snack

Yogurt with Berries

- **Preparation Time: 5 minutes**

- **Ingredients:**

  - 1/2 cup Greek yogurt

  - 1/4 cup mixed berries (blueberries, raspberries)

- **Directions**:

  1. Serve Greek yogurt with mixed berries.

- Nutrition Value per Serving: Calories: 150 kcal | Protein: 12g | Carbs: 20g | Fat: 3g | Fiber: 3g

Week 2: Day 13

Breakfast

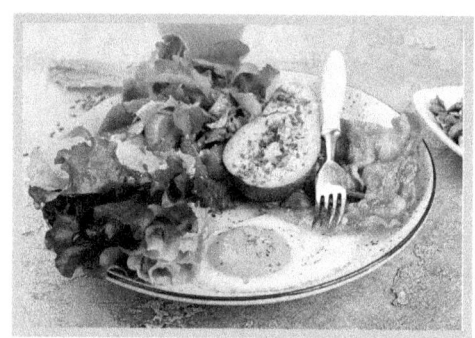

Avocado Toast with Poached Egg

- Preparation Time: 15 minutes

- Ingredients:

- 1 piece of toasted whole wheat bread

- 1/2 avocado, mashed

- 1 poached egg

- 1 teaspoon chopped fresh cilantro

- Salt and pepper to taste

- **Directions:**

1. Top toasted whole wheat bread with mashed avocado.

2. Place a poached egg on top.

3. Sprinkle with chopped cilantro, salt, and pepper.

- **Nutrition Value per Serving:** Calories: 250 kcal | Protein: 10g | Carbs: 15g | Fat: 15g | Fiber: 6g

Lunch

Spinach and Mushroom Omelette

- **Preparation Time: 20 minutes**

- **Ingredients:**

  - 3 eggs

  - 1/4 cup baby spinach

  - 1/4 cup sliced mushrooms

- 2 tablespoons diced red bell pepper

- 1 tablespoon shredded mozzarella cheese

- 1 teaspoon olive oil

- Salt and pepper to taste

- **Directions**:

1. Beat eggs with salt and pepper in a bowl.

2. In a non-stick pan, heat olive oil.

3. Add baby spinach, sliced mushrooms, and diced red bell pepper. Sauté until tender.

4. Pour beaten eggs into the pan. Cook until set.

5. Sprinkle shredded mozzarella cheese on one half of the omelette, then fold the other half over.

- Nutrition Value per Serving: Calories: 280 kcal | Protein: 20g | Carbs: 5g | Fat: 20g | Fiber: 2g

Dinner

Baked Cod with Lemon and Herbs

- **Preparation Time: 25 minutes**

- **Ingredients:**

  - 4 oz cod fillet

  - 1 tablespoon olive oil

  - 1 tablespoon lemon juice

  - 1/2 teaspoon dried thyme

  - 1/4 teaspoon garlic powder

  - Lemon slices for garnish

  - Salt and pepper to taste

- **Directions:**

  1. Preheat the oven. Cod fillet should be put on a baking pan.

  2. Garnish with lemon juice and olive oil.

3. Sprinkle with dried thyme, garlic powder, salt, and pepper.

4. Top with lemon slices.

5. Bake until the cod flakes easily with a fork.

- **Nutrition Value per Serving:** Calories: 220 kcal | Protein: 25g | Carbs: 1g | Fat: 12g | Fiber: 0g

Snack

Mixed Nuts

- Preparation Time: 5 minutes

- Ingredients:

- 1/4 cup mixed nuts (almonds, cashews, walnuts)

- Directions:

1. Serve mixed nuts as a snack.

Nutrition Value per Serving:

Calories: 200 kcal

Protein: 5g

Carbs: 6g

Fat: 18g

Fiber: 3g

Week 2: Day 14

Breakfast

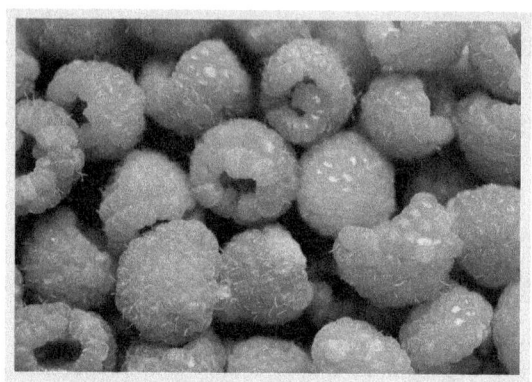

Berry Smoothie

- Preparation Time: 10 minutes

- Ingredients:

- Berry mixture of blueberries, strawberries, and raspberries, 1/2 cup

- 1/2 banana

- 1/2 cup unsweetened almond milk

- 1/2 cup Greek yogurt

- 1 tablespoon chia seeds

- **Directions:**

1. Blend mixed berries, banana, almond milk, Greek yogurt, and chia seeds until smooth.

- **Nutrition Value per Serving:** Calories: 250 kcal | Protein: 10g | Carbs: 40g | Fat: 6g | Fiber: 10g

Lunch

Quinoa Salad with Roasted Vegetables

- **Preparation Time: 30 minutes**

- **Ingredients:**

- 1/2 cup cooked quinoa

- 1/4 cup roasted mixed vegetables (bell peppers, zucchini, onions)

- 2 tablespoons crumbled feta cheese

- 1 tablespoon chopped fresh parsley

- 1 tablespoon balsamic vinegar

- 1 tablespoon olive oil

- Salt and pepper to taste

- **Directions:**

1. In a bowl, combine cooked quinoa, roasted mixed vegetables, crumbled f

eta cheese, chopped parsley, balsamic vinegar, olive oil, salt, and pepper.

- Nutrition Value per Serving:

Calories: 280 kcal | Protein: 10g | Carbs: 30g | Fat: 15g | Fiber: 6g

Dinner

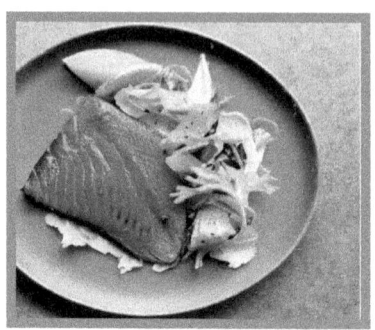

Vegetable Stir-Fry with Tofu

- Preparation Time: 30 minutes

- Ingredients:

- 1/2 cup firm tofu, cubed

- 1 cup mixed vegetables, including bell peppers, broccoli, and carrots)

- 2 tablespoons low-sodium soy sauce

- 1 tablespoon hoisin sauce

- 1 teaspoon sesame oil

- 1/2 teaspoon minced garlic

- 1/2 teaspoon minced ginger

- Sliced green onions for garnish

- Directions

1. In a pan, heat sesame oil. Cook the diced tofu until browned.

2. Add mixed vegetables and sauté until tender.

3. Stir in low-sodium soy sauce, hoisin sauce, minced garlic, and minced ginger.

4. Garnish with sliced green onions.

- **Nutrition Value per Serving:** Calories: 300 kcal | Protein: 15g | Carbs: 30g | Fat: 15g | Fiber: 6g

Snack

Cottage Cheese with Peaches

- Preparation Time: 5 minutes

- Ingredients:

- 1/2 cup low-fat cottage cheese

- 1/4 cup sliced peaches (fresh or canned)

- Directions:

1. Serve low-fat cottage cheese with sliced peaches.

- Nutrition Value per Serving: Calories: 150 kcal | Protein: 12g | Carbs: 15g | Fat: 4g | Fiber: 2g

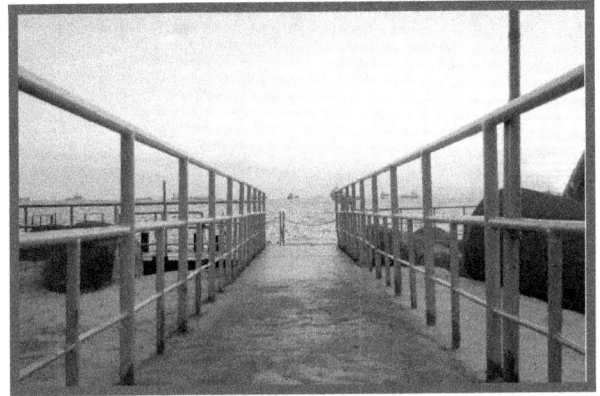

Week 3: Day 15

Memory-Enhancing Meals

Breakfast

Veggie Omelette

- **Preparation Time: 20 minutes**

- **Ingredients:**

  - 3 eggs

  - 1/4 cup diced bell peppers

  - 1/4 cup diced tomatoes

  - 1/4 cup diced zucchini

  - 1/4 cup chopped spinach

  - 1 tablespoon of freshly chopped herbs, such as parsley and chives

  - Salt and pepper to taste

- **Directions**:

1. Eggs should be beaten with salt and pepper in a bowl.

2. In a non-stick pan, sauté diced bell peppers, diced tomatoes, diced zucchini, and chopped spinach until tender.

3. Pour beaten eggs into the pan. Cook until set.

4. Sprinkle with chopped fresh herbs.

- **Nutrition Value per Serving:** Calories: 250 kcal | Protein: 18g | Carbs: 10g | Fat: 15g | Fiber: 3g

Lunch

Lentil Soup

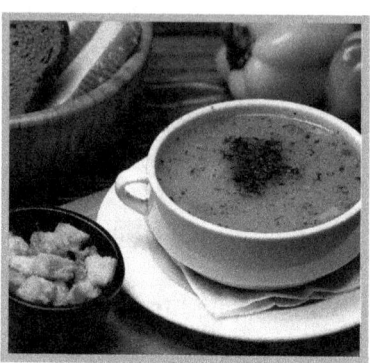

- Preparation Time: 40 minutes

- Ingredients:

  - 1/2 cup cooked lentils

  - 1/4 cup diced carrots

  - 1/4 cup diced celery

  - 1/4 cup diced onion

  - 2 cups low-sodium vegetable broth

  - 1/2 teaspoon ground cumin

  - 1/4 teaspoon dried thyme

- Salt and pepper to taste

- **Directions**:

1. In a pot, sauté diced carrots, diced celery, and diced onion until tender.

2. Add cooked lentils, low-sodium vegetable broth, ground cumin, dried thyme, salt, and pepper.

3. Simmer until flavors meld.

- Nutrition Value per Serving: Calories: 220 kcal | Protein: 10g | Carbs: 40g | Fat: 1g | Fiber: 10g

Dinner

Grilled Shrimp with Asparagus

- Preparation Time: 25 minutes

Ingredients:

- 4 ounces of peeled and deveined shrimp

- 1/2 bunch asparagus, trimmed

- 1 tablespoon olive oil

- 1 teaspoon lemon juice

- 1/2 teaspoon dried dill

- Salt and pepper to taste

- Directions:

1. Preheat the grill. Toss shrimp and asparagus with olive oil, lemon juice, dried dill, salt, and pepper.

2. Grill until shrimp are opaque and asparagus is tender.-

Nutrition Value per Serving: Calories: 200 kcal | Protein: 25g | Carbs: 5g | Fat: 10g | Fiber: 2g

Week 3: Day 16

Breakfast

Overnight Chia Pudding

- **Preparation Time: 10 minutes (plus overnight chilling)**

- **Ingredients**:

    - 1/4 cup chia seeds

    - 1 cup unsweetened almond milk

    - 1/2 teaspoon vanilla extract

    - 1/2 banana, sliced

    - 1 tablespoon of walnuts and almonds, sliced

- **Directions**:

    1. In a bowl, mix chia seeds, almond milk, and vanilla extract.

    2. Cover

and refrigerate overnight.

3. In the morning, layer chia pudding with sliced banana and chopped nuts.

- Nutrition Value per Serving: Calories: 300 kcal | Protein: 8g | Carbs: 25g | Fat: 20g | Fiber: 10g

Lunch

Tofu and Vegetable Stir-Fry

- **Preparation Time: 30 minutes**

- **Ingredients:**

  - 1/2 cup firm tofu, cubed

  - 1 cup mixed vegetables (broccoli, snap peas, carrots)

  - 2 tablespoons low-sodium soy sauce

  - 1 tablespoon hoisin sauce

  - 1 tablespoon sesame oil

  - 1/2 teaspoon minced garlic

  - 1/2 teaspoon minced ginger

  - Sliced green onions for garnish

- **Directions:**

  1. In a pan, heat sesame oil. Cook the diced tofu until browned.

2. Add mixed vegetables and sauté until tender.

3. Stir in low-sodium soy sauce, hoisin sauce, minced garlic, and minced ginger.

4. Garnish with sliced green onions.

- **Nutrition Value per Serving:** Calories: 250 kcal | Protein: 15g | Carbs: 20g | Fat: 15g | Fiber: 6g

Dinner

Herb-Roasted Chicken with Steamed Broccoli

- **Preparation Time: 40 minutes**

- **Ingredients:**

  - 4 oz chicken breast

  - 1 tablespoon olive oil

  - 1/2 teaspoon dried rosemary

  - 1/4 teaspoon dried thyme

- 1/4 teaspoon garlic powder

- 1/4 teaspoon onion powder

- Salt and pepper to taste

- Steamed broccoli for serving

- **Directions**:

1. Preheat the oven. Put a baking sheet with chicken breast on it.

2. Drizzle with olive oil and sprinkle with dried rosemary, dried thyme, garlic powder, onion powder, salt, and pepper.

3. Bake the chicken for the recommended time.

4. Serve with steamed broccoli.

- **Nutrition Value per Serving:** Calories: 250 kcal | Protein: 30g | Carbs: 5g | Fat: 10g | Fiber: 2g

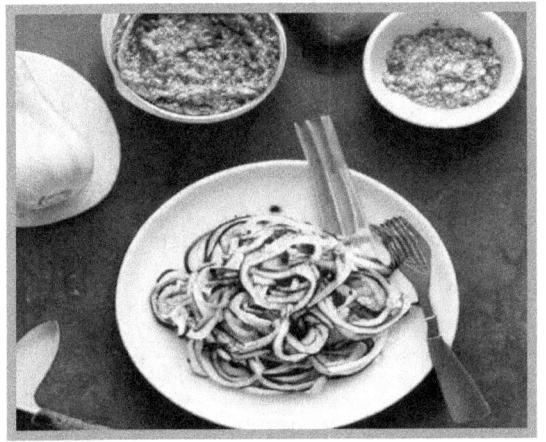

Week 3: Day 17

Breakfast - Whole Grain Waffles

- **Preparation Time: 25 minutes**

- **Ingredients:**

  - 1 whole grain waffle

  - A half-cup of mixed berries (strawberries, blueberries).

  - 1 tablespoon of finely chopped nuts (walnuts, almonds) - 1 teaspoon honey

- Directions:

  1. Toast whole grain waffle according to package instructions.

  2. Top with mixed berries, chopped nuts, and honey.

- **Nutrition Value per Serving:** Calories: 250 kcal | Protein: 5g | Carbs: 40g | Fat: 10g | Fiber: 6g

Lunch

Chickpea and Spinach Salad

- Preparation Time: 20 minutes

- Ingredients:

- Drained and washed half a cup of canned chickpeas

- 1 cup baby spinach

- 1/4 cup diced cucumber

- 1/4 cup diced red onion

- 2 tablespoons crumbled feta cheese

- 1 tablespoon chopped fresh dill

- 1 tablespoon olive oil

- 1 tablespoon lemon juice

- Salt and pepper to taste

- Directions:

1. In a bowl, combine chickpeas, baby spinach, diced cucumber, diced red onion, crumbled feta cheese, chopped fresh dill, olive oil, lemon juice, salt, and pepper.

- **Nutrition Value per Serving:** Calories: 280 kcal | Protein: 10g | Carbs: 30g | Fat: 15g | Fiber: 8g

Dinner

Turkey Meatballs with Marinara Sauce

- **Preparation Time: 40 minutes**

- **Ingredients:**

  - 4 turkey meatballs (about 4 oz)

  - 1/2 cup low-sodium marinara sauce

  - 50% of a cooked serving of whole-wheat spaghetti

  - 1 tablespoon grated Parmesan cheese

  - Fresh basil leaves for garnish

- **Directions**:

1. Preheat the oven. Bake turkey meatballs according to package instructions.

2. Heat marinara sauce and serve with cooked whole wheat spaghetti.

3. Top with turkey meatballs, grated Parmesan cheese, and fresh basil leaves.

- **Nutrition Value per Serving:** Calories: 320 kcal | Protein: 20g | Carbs: 30g | Fat: 12g | Fiber: 6g

Week 3: Day 18

Breakfast - Scrambled Eggs with Spinach

- **Preparation Time: 15 minutes**

- **Ingredients:**

  - 3 eggs

  - 1/4 cup chopped spinach

  - 1 tablespoon diced red bell pepper

  - 1 tablespoon diced red onion

  - 1 tablespoon crumbled feta cheese

  - Salt and pepper to taste

- **Directions:**

  1. Stir salt and pepper into beaten eggs in a bowl

  2. In a non-stick pan, sauté chopped spinach, diced red bell pepper, and diced red onion until tender.

  3. Pour beaten eggs into the pan. Cook until set.

  4. Sprinkle it with crumbled feta cheese.

Nutrition Value per Serving:

Calories: 250 kcal

Protein: 18g

Carbs: 5g

Fat: 18g

Fiber: 2g.

Lunch

Mediterranean Wrap

- Preparation Time: 20 minutes

- Ingredients:

- 1 whole wheat tortilla

- 1/4 cup hummus

- 1/4 cup chopped cucumber

- 1/4 cup chopped tomato

- 1/4 cup chopped red onion

- 2 tablespoons crumbled feta cheese

- 1 tablespoon chopped fresh parsley

- Directions:

1. Spread hummus on the whole wheat tortilla.

2. Top with chopped cucumber, chopped tomato, chopped red onion, crumbled feta cheese, and chopped fresh parsley.

3. Roll up the tortilla into a wrap.

Nutrition Value per Serving: Calories: 300 kcal

Protein: 10g

Carbs: 35g |

Fat: 15g |

Fiber: 6g

Dinner

Salmon with Quinoa and Steamed Broccoli

- **Preparation Time: 30 minutes**

- **Ingredients:**

  - 4 oz salmon fillet

  - 1/2 cup cooked quinoa

  - Steamed broccoli for serving

  - Lemon wedge for garnish

  - Salt and pepper to taste

- **Directions:**

  1. Preheat the oven. Place salmon fillet on a baking sheet.

  2. Bake until salmon flakes easily with a fork.

  3. Serve with cooked quinoa, steamed broccoli, and a lemon wedge.

Nutrition Value per Serving:

Calories: 300 kcal |

Protein: 25g |

Carbs: 25g |

Fat: 12g |

Fiber: 4g

Week 3: Day 19

Breakfast

Peanut Butter Banana Toast

- **Preparation Time: 10 minutes**

- **Ingredients:**

  - 1 piece of toasted whole wheat bread

  - 2 tablespoons natural peanut butter

  - 1/2 banana, sliced

  - 1 teaspoon honey

- **Directions:**

  1. Spread natural peanut butter on toasted whole wheat bread.

  2. Top with sliced banana and drizzle with honey.

- Nutrition Value per Serving: Calories: 300 kcal | Protein: 8g | Carbs: 35g | Fat: 15g | Fiber: 6g

Lunch

Tomato and Mozzarella Salad

- **Preparation Time: 10 minutes**

- **Ingredients:**

  - 1 medium tomato, sliced

  - ounces of sliced fresh mozzarella cheese

  - 1/4 cup fresh basil leaves

  - 1 tablespoon balsamic vinegar

  - 1 tablespoon olive oil

  - Salt and pepper to taste

- **Directions:**

  1. Arrange tomato and mozzarella slices on a plate.

  2. Top with fresh basil leaves.

  3. Add a drizzle of olive oil and balsamic vinegar.

- **Nutrition Value per Serving:** Calories: 250 kcal | Protein: 10g | Carbs: 5g | Fat: 20g | Fiber: 1g

Dinner

Baked Zucchini Boats

- **Preparation Time: 35 minutes**

- **Ingredients:**

  - 2 small zucchinis, halved lengthwise

  - 1/2 cup cooked quinoa

  - 1/4 cup diced tomatoes

  - 1/4 cup diced bell pepper

  - 2 tablespoons shredded mozzarella cheese

  - 1 tablespoon chopped fresh parsley

  - 1 teaspoon olive oil

  - 1/4 teaspoon dried oregano

  - Salt and pepper to taste

- **Directions**:

1. Preheat the oven. Scoop out the center of zucchini halves to create a boat shape.

2. In a bowl, mix cooked quinoa, diced tomatoes, diced bell pepper, shredded mozzarella cheese, chopped fresh parsley, olive oil, dried oregano, salt, and pepper.

3. Stuff zucchini halves with quinoa mixture.

4. Bake until zucchini is tender and the filling is heated through.

- **Nutrition Value per Serving**: Calories: 300 kcal | Protein: 15g | Carbs: 30g | Fat: 12g | Fiber: 6g

WEEK 3: DAY 20

Breakfast

Breakfast Burrito

- Preparation Time: 20 minutes

- Ingredients:

- 1 whole wheat tortilla

- 2 eggs, scrambled

- 1/4 cup washed and rinsed black beans

- 1/4 avocado, sliced

- 2 tablespoons salsa

- Salt and pepper to taste

- Directions:

1. Fill a whole wheat tortilla with scrambled eggs, black beans, avocado slices, salsa, salt, and pepper.

2. Roll up the tortilla into a burrito.

- **Nutrition Value per Serving**:

Calories: 350 kcal |

Protein: 18g |

Carbs: 30g |

Fat: 18g |

Fiber: 10g

Lunch

Greek Yogurt with Cucumber

- **Preparation Time: 5 minutes**

- **Ingredients:**

  - 1/2 cup Greek yogurt

  - 1/4 cup diced cucumber

- **Directions:**

  1. Serve Greek yogurt with diced cucumber.

- **Nutrition Value per Serving**: Calories: 150 kcal | Protein: 15g | Carbs: 10g | Fat: 6g | Fiber: 2g

Dinner

Apple Slices with Cheese

- **Preparation Time: 5 minutes**

- **Ingredients:**

  - 1 small apple, sliced

  - 1 oz cheese (cheddar, mozzarella)

- **Directions**:

  1. Serve apple slices with cheese.

- **Nutrition Value per Serving:** Calories: 200 kcal | Protein: 8g | Carbs: 20g | Fat: 10g | Fiber: 4g

Week 3 Day 21

Sustaining Mental Clarity

Breakfast

Rice Cakes with Almond Butter

- **Preparation Time: 5 minutes**

- **Ingredients:**

  - 2 rice cakes

  - 2 tablespoons almond butter

- **Directions:**

  1. Spread almond butter on rice cakes.

- **Nutrition Value per Serving:** Calories: 200 kcal |
Protein: 5g | Carbs: 20g | Fat: 12g | Fiber: 3g

Lunch

Hummus with Bell Pepper Slices

- Preparation Time: 5 minutes

- Ingredients:

  - 1/4 cup hummus

  - 1 small bell pepper, sliced

- Directions:

  1. Serve hummus with bell pepper slices for dipping.

- Nutrition Value per Serving: Calories: 150 kcal | Protein: 4g | Carbs: 15g | Fat: 10g | Fiber: 5g

Dinner

Mixed Berries with Cottage Cheese

- **Preparation Time: 5 minutes**

- **Ingredients:**

  - Berry mixture of blueberries, raspberries, and strawberries, 1/2 cup

  - 1/4 cup low-fat cottage cheese

- **Directions:**

  1. Serve mixed berries with low-fat cottage cheese.

- Nutrition Value per Serving: Calories: 150 kcal | Protein: 10g | Carbs: 20g | Fat: 3g | Fiber: 6g.

Enjoy your delicious and nutritious meals throughout the third week of your meal plan journey! Remember, these recipes are just a starting point, and you can always add your own twists and variations to make them uniquely yours.

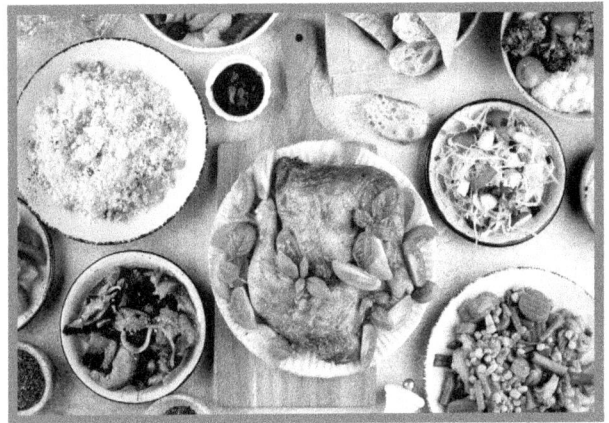

Lifestyle Tips for Optimal Brain Health

Maintaining a healthy brain isn't just about what you eat; it's also about how you live. Here are three essential lifestyle tips to keep your brain sharp:

Exercise, Hydration, and Stress Management

1. Exercise Regularly: Physical activity isn't just good for your body; it's great for your brain too. Regular exercise increases blood flow to the brain, encourages the growth of new brain cells, and enhances cognitive function. Aim for at least 150 minutes of moderate-intensity aerobic exercise each week, like brisk walking or swimming.

2. Stay Hydrated: Dehydration can lead to cognitive impairment, affecting memory and concentration. Ensure you drink enough water

throughout the day to keep your brain hydrated. A good rule of thumb is to aim for eight 8-ounce glasses of water daily, but individual needs may vary.

3. Manage Stress: Chronic stress can have a detrimental impact on brain health. Practice stress management techniques such as mindfulness, meditation, or yoga to reduce stress levels. Adequate sleep is also crucial, as it allows your brain to recover and consolidate memories.

Incorporating these lifestyle tips into your daily routine can help safeguard your cognitive function and promote overall brain health.

Measuring Chart for Converting Recipes

Tools for Liquid Measurements

"For precise liquid measurements, equip yourself with essential tools: KitchenAid's 3-piece Measuring Cup Set, available at Wayfair for $29.99, and a stainless steel measuring spoon set from Crate & Barrel, priced at $12.95. The liquid measuring cups come in clear glass or plastic and offer capacities of 1, 2, 4, or 8 cups, complete with incremental markings, handles, and spouts for effortless pouring. Remember, never use dry measuring cups for liquids or vice versa, as this may lead to inaccurate measurements. Opt for nested measuring spoons instead, offering ¼ teaspoon, ½ teaspoon, 1 teaspoon, and 1 tablespoon measures, versatile for both dry and liquid ingredients."

measuring tools boast both metric and standard markings, you're all set; otherwise, this liquid measurement chart will save the day.

0.5 ml = ⅛ teaspoon

1 ml = ¼ teaspoon

2 ml = 1/3 teaspoon

5 ml = 1 teaspoon

15 ml = 1 tablespoon

25 ml = 1 tablespoon + 2 teaspoons

50 ml equates to two liquid ounces, or one-fourth of a cup.

75 milliliters is equivalent to three liquid ounces, or one third of a cup.

125 ml is equal to 4 liquid ounces, or 12 cup.

150 ml equates to 5 liquid ounces, or 2 1/3 cups.

6 fluid ounces or 3/4 cup equals 175 ml.

250 ml = eight ounces of liquid = 1 cup 500 ml = 1 pint = 2 cups

1 liter is equal to 1 quart, 2 pints, and 4 cups.

Converting metric measurements to U.S. measurements is a breeze with this handy guide. Prepare your culinary delights without a hitch, and embrace the joy of cooking with precision!

Accurate measuring is the key to perfect results in your culinary endeavors. To measure liquids correctly, set your liquid measuring cup on a level surface and pour in the liquid. To ensure precision, bend down and align your eyes with the markings on the cup's side; avoid eyeballing it from above as it may deceive you.

In baking, precise measurements are paramount, as too much or too little liquid can impact the recipe's outcome. Exceptionally for small quantities, like 1 tablespoon or less, fill the appropriate measuring spoon to the rim without any spills.

Keep these liquid measurement charts handy for seamless cooking. While memorizing some conversions can be helpful (e.g., 3 teaspoons = 1 tablespoon), double-checking is always wise for perfect results. With this comprehensive guide by your side, you'll effortlessly master the art of accurate measuring. Happy cooking!

Conclusion

More than merely a cookbook, "Alzheimer's Cookbook for Seniors" offers hope to people dealing with cognitive impairment. We've looked at a variety of delectable dishes that are created to energize the body and the mind within these pages.

This recipe serves as an example of how it's possible to be upbeat despite having Alzheimer's. We empower ourselves and our loved ones to embrace a life of fulfillment via well chosen ingredients and well-balanced, delicious cuisine.

It's not just about eating; it's also about creating enduring memories, spending time with others, and appreciating each bite. This cuisine emphasizes the strength of the human spirit and the significant role that diet plays in cognitive health.

Let's keep in mind that taking care of our bodies and minds are equally important as we get to the end of our delicious trip. Whatever the difficulties we face, together we can cherish every second and set out on a path to happiness, well-being, and a life lived to the fullest.

Share your feedback and inspire other readers by leaving a positive review.

Have a Joyful Cooking Experience!

WEEKLY MEAL PLANNER

DATE ——————

MONDAY	BREAKFAST		
	LUNCH		
	DINNER		
TUESDAY	BREAKFAST		
	LUNCH		
	DINNER		
WEDNESDAY	BREAKFAST		
	LUNCH		
	DINNER		
THURSDAY	BREAKFAST		
	LUNCH		
	DINNER		
FRIDAY	BREAKFAST		
	LUNCH		
	DINNER		
SATURDAY	BREAKFAST		
	LUNCH		
	DINNER		
SUNDAY	BREAKFAST		
	LUNCH		
	DINNER		

APPETIZERS AND SNACKS

PHYSICAL ACTIVITIES

NOTES